My Journe

Metastatic

Text Copyright © 2018 Lavinia Urban

All rights reserved

ISBN: 9781980407706
Imprint: Independently published

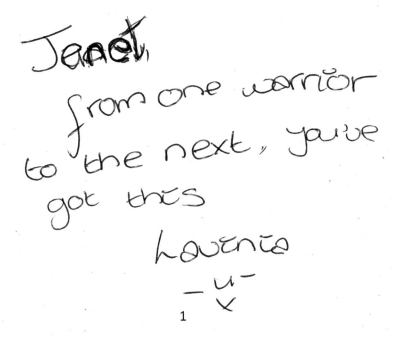

Janet,
from one warrior
to the next, you've
got this
                Lavinia
                  -u-
                   X

Disclaimer

This book is my real-life retelling of my battle with cancer, that started in 2017. I talk openly and, in some cases, in graphic detail. If you are offended easily then this is not the book for you.

Message from Editor

This book is not perfectly edited. There is a level of "raw-ness" to what she has to say that would be lost in a perfectly edited book. Misspelled words have been corrected, missing punctuation has been fixed. This is a journal of one person's experience with her most recent fight against metastatic cancer. Although this was written with the intent to be published, this is not a novel and should not be treated as such. This is Lavinia's story of the journey, she, her husband, and her children took this past year as she fought cancer. Her experiences in her own words. There is an honesty seldom found anywhere outside of a private journal. You cannot read this and walk away untouched by her fight this past year. She truly is a survivor.

Joyce Wetherbee, Editor.

Early days (before cancer.)

I've always been a fighter from as far back as I can remember. There was the time when I was around three years old and thinking that I was some type of superhero. I'd climbed out of my third storey bedroom window before fear set in and I grabbed hold of the window and screamed as I dangled there. Problem was that my mother is deaf so couldn't hear me. It was our neighbour who came running and saved me.

Then there were the years of abuse at the hands of my mother, then in later years my brother joined in too.

There were also the times that I was back and forth into foster care.

Then back in 2000 I was given two hours to live with my appendix followed by two weeks to live when that got infected.

Each of those things have sculpted me into the person I am today. They made me a cautious, untrusting, distant, insecure person. It was only after meeting my husband that I slowly mellowed. He was my knight in shining armour, and still is. He is the one person who always has my back and pushes me to be all that I can be – my own personal cheerleader.

Our life grew stronger with each second. We had two daughters before we married then in 2012 I published my first book. Who was the first person to congratulate me and support me whilst others had no faith? You guessed it.

Our life together was going great. I was even diagnosed with fibromyalgia but that was a blip and something we could cope with. Then in the middle of March 2017 I noticed that my areola on my left breast was slightly raised. I showed my husband and he said that maybe it was because of my time of month. *Yeah he was probably right* I'd thought and thought nothing of it. If anything I thought it had shrunk or rather gone back to normal but then towards the end of month i noticed it again and this time felt worried abs my husband said I should make a doctor's appointment. He told me not to worry as it was probably a cyst like our fifteen year old just had.

So on the 3rd April, the day before my birthday, I headed to the doctors. I expected her to send me to the hospital to get it drained because it was a cyst but she told me that she was concerned and didn't think that it was a cyst. She told me that she would send a referral to the hospital and I should hear something within two weeks.

Worry sat heavy but I had my birthday and that weekend I was going to at an author signing event in Chester. I just needed to put it out of my mind.

The day we travelled down (7th April) an appointment letter arrived in the post that morning. I was one sleep closer go finding out what this was.

2017

27th April

This was the day of the appointment. By this time the lump was slightly bigger and I had pain in the right side of my breast, causing difficulty for me to sleep on that side. Annoying when that is the one side that I slept better.

The doctor who saw me was baffled by my areola and it wasn't until feeling my breast and hearing me cry out that she became suspicious. She pressed in my armpit and said that she had noticed a few lumps in there which are my lymph nodes but nothing that would worry her but it is best if I went down to the mammogram department and have some tests.

Three mammograms, one ultrasound, two biopsies and two markers placed inside my breast, followed by a nurse placing her body weight on the places where the biopsies had been taken. It left me in lots of pain and feeling emotional. I learned that one shot of local anaesthetic is never enough for me because I still felt the first device go into my breast. This resulted in them quickly giving me more local anaesthetic.

I was told that the bit near my areola does look like cancer. My lymph nodes look swollen on both sides so that could mean I have systematic arthritis but as I have fibromyalgia and that is systematic then it could just be that.

I was told to come back the following Thursday, 4th May, for the results. Now I live my life by trying to think positively so I had wrapped my head around it being nothing to worry about. Plus, I was getting the results on Star Wars day so that was a positive sign... wasn't it?

4th May

Leading up to this day I was in a lot of pain from the mammograms but I was thinking positively. I had have had trouble sleeping properly and have had to resort to propping pillows and blankets on either side of me so that I do not roll onto my breast. My husband has resorted to sleeping on the sofa as he does not want to disturb me or roll into me whilst sleeping.

When I first arrived I was told that my results were locked so go grab a coffee then come back. I did.

When we went back I was told straight that I had a tumour measuring less than 2cm and the lymph nodes are cancerous so I need to undergo a series of tests to check them out.

I still felt positive even though my husband felt as though someone had sucker punched him. He told the doctor that he felt as though he had the hand of death. The times when he had tried to reassure people that their loved ones would be okay but they hadn't. He took those to heart and blamed himself. I told him that I never wanted to hear that because I am not going to die. I refuse to.

That day we were introduced to our cancer nurse. She was lovely but I was nervous and I wouldn't shut up. I am a nervous talker and I own it.

The nurse was lovely though she explained that she would be right beside me through my journey. Then she took my blood before showing us to ultrasound where they scanned my liver.

All clear that doctor had said and I felt my smile grow.

Then it was on to x-ray where they x-rayed my chest.

Then it was time to go to nuclear science. I had forgotten that I was told that a guide would show me around. They do tell you that the day you find out you have cancer there is this fog. I have to say that I agree to an extent. Somethings were crystal clear whereas others are a blur. I even lost some of my paperwork when I got home.

At nuclear science they injected me with radioactive dye and told me to come back in two hours. My husband used that time to take me to the beach. It was nice to just sit there and try not to think about the crap going on in my life.

The job of this test was to scan my bones. The downside was the fact that I wasn't allowed to hug my ten year old daughter for 24 hours.

Before leaving the hospital I had called my Nan and told her the news before texting one of my aunts just as another texted me, after having received a call from my Nan.

I was numb though. It was easy to text what I had heard but not so easy to speak it.

On the way home we had decided to tell our daughter's. I didn't expect it to be right away but when we had arrived home my husband had told the girls that they had to stay an arm's length distance away from me because of a test I had had. Our eldest wanted to know details, or rather she wanted to cut to the chase as to whether I had cancer or not.

My husband confirmed it. All the while I said nothing.

My youngest began to sob and instantly I had to walk away and go into the other room. It was the first time I had allowed myself to cry but after ten seconds I had chastised myself. I told myself that there was nothing to cry about. It's a tiny bit of cancer and they will cut it out so we could move on with our lives.

Our eldest was too concerned with the fact that she had exams. At first it took me by surprise but I realised that this is her way of dealing with things.

The next day my husband went to work and our eldest went for her exam leaving me alone with the youngest. That morning seemed to drag. We kept looking at that clock and willing 1pm to come around, as that would be 24 hours from the radioactive dye was injected.

As soon as that clock turned to 1pm we hugged each other as best as my body would allow – my right side was still sore.

9ᵗʰ May

This was the day I was back at the hospital. I was told that we would arrive at 11am, the same time as everyone else, and be called when ready.

We arrive half an hour early. Not only that, our eldest daughter had come along. She seemed to be struggling to process everything. The day before I'd caught her sending a message to her friend informing her that I am dying and she didn't care. Obviously she did care but was struggling and had asked if she could come to the hospital with me and her dad.

Arriving early at the hospital I didn't expect to get called in early but I did and was introduced to my surgeon. I expected this to be positive. He was going to operate on me and I would be good but then he started talking about my lymph nodes being cancerous and how there is a part of my skull that has cancer and how they are suspicious of a lymph node buried deep in my chest.

All this being said and I could feel my positivity is ebbing away. I felt sick. It was as though I was inside a fish tank with everyone looking in.

"Is it curable?" I found myself asking.

Both the surgeon and nurse looked at each other before finally the surgeon spoke. He told me that it is not curable but it is treatable.

My heart stopped. A part of me, a huge part, wanted to cry. I wanted to kick, scream and bawl like a baby. But as I glanced around I saw my fifteen year old daughter sitting there, unsure of what to do. I saw my husband, who looked as if he was about to break and was struggling to be strong for me.

Quickly I looked away. I couldn't allow my family to be sad. I couldn't allow the doctor to look at me with pity, not that he stopped. I had to be strong. I needed to pull myself together and fight this.

I am a fighter. It was what I was born to do. Life only gives you what you can handle so I know that I had to be a ninja. A ninja with a huge fucking smile on my face. I also knew that I needed to be positive both inside and out. And honestly, it took a few days for that to happen. I didn't cry though. I refused to.

Leading up to this day I was smoking one to four cigarettes a day. Yes the cancer may not be in my lungs but I looked at the reality of it. I heard my granddads words screaming in my head. So many times, before he passed away, he would tell me to quit. I had quit through every pregnancy but afterwards I always went back. But not that day. That day I said 'no more.'

15th May

I went to see my oncologist specialist and discovered that this Dr specialised in chemotherapy. He had a plan but he also informed me that they were unsure of what exactly was causing the abnormalities on my lymph nodes and skull were. I had a complete 'huh?' moment. He had a plan though. He wanted to start me off with 18 to 24 weeks of chemo which would be administered every three weeks. After the first four sessions they would see if my skull and lymph nodes reacted to that. That way they can see whether they need to do something else or whether they are something other than cancer.

Honestly I left the Dr on a high that we were finally about to kick arse but confused because they were confused.

I was also informed that it is hereditary. Even though I only know of one person in my family who's had it and that was my maternal grandfather's sister who died when I was young, maybe before I was born, after losing her battle with breast cancer for the third time.

According to the Dr if there have been at least two women under the age of forty who have had it then it is hereditary and who's to say that I don't have cousins, great cousins etc who've had it. Apparently it also means that prostate cancer is highly likely in men too.

Leaving the Drs office we were escorted into the main waiting room by a nurse. Apparently this was my new nurse. This nurse specialised in breast cancer that has spread and even though they are not 100% sure about the lymph nodes and skull they wanted to give me a new nurse. This nurse is classed as a secondary breast cancer nurse.

Now don't get me wrong here, the nurse was nice but when I told her that I am going to have fun trying on wigs she became a bit of a party pooper by telling me all the ways it would not be fun whilst I stared at her with a vacant expression whilst trying to smile.

This journey is mine and I am trying to be positive. I did not want to deal with any type of negativity so we made our excuses and left. She did however tell me to go ahead and make a wig appointment before I lose my hair so the specialist knows what my current style is.

18th May

Today I announced to my friends on Facebook that I have cancer. Here is what I put along with the image.

"Hi everyone. I have been toying with making this status for a long time but in all honesty I was not in the right frame of mind. I am not saying that I am now but I am definitely stronger and over the last couple of months I have been wanting to make statuses but deleting them. I could have continued on and kept it quiet but there will be times when I am feeling down and I want to cry and rant on FB, in a hope that people can say something funny to pick me up.

I have cancer and even though it is not curable, it is treatable. I am a very strong and positive person so I know I can fight this. The biggest reason for me posting this is because I have had invites to attend events, in the next couple of months, and I feel bad saying that I can't but not being able to give the real reason. I have also had readers asking when my next books are out, etc. But as you can imagine, my mind has been elsewhere.

In October I am due to sign at The Darker Side of Fiction in Peterborough, right now this is up in the air. My chemo starts in a couple of weeks and will last 18 to 24 weeks. The specialists think that I could still attend but that all depends on how I am during the treatment. So it is one of those 'watch this space' situations. I really want to go to the event though and Rachel and Jo are well aware of what is going on.

The Edinburgh event I will be hosting next year will still be going ahead though.

Thank you for reading and sorry it was long."

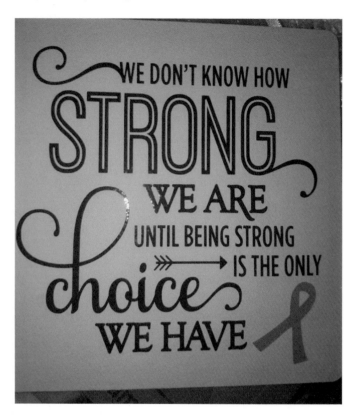

Because I had the confidence to write this post I was now able to share the image of my charm bracelet. I plan that before the year is out I will have another charm that says I am a 2017 breast cancer survivor.

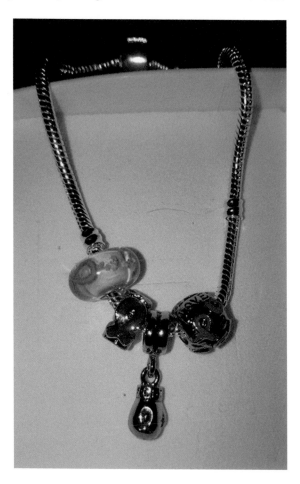

22nd May

I went for a wig appointment. I was told to get this measured up beforehand so the specialist could see what my hair looks like before I lose it. I had fun with this. I tried on all different types and colours and discovered that I do not suit blonde hair.

24th May

More bloods and a CT scan. I had to arrive an hour early for the CT scan and drink this yucky stuff which I mixed with orange cordial. Then I went for the scan and I wasn't told that I will get a sensation that I will wet myself. I discovered this for myself and it was not a nice feeling.

25th May

With chemo coming up I wanted something inspirational to put on my bedroom wall so that every morning and every night I would see this.

It is a quote by Albus Dumbledore from Harry Potter.

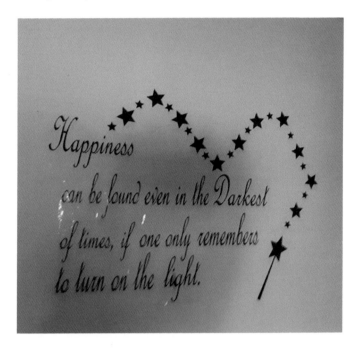

29th May

Today I had my bloods taken, saw my oncologist, and had a heart scan. Made status asking what funny books to download. Was told that the cancer is also in my chest bone and lymph nodes there. Or rather they are almost 100% sure that that is what it is. I think I wanted to be sick when the consultant told me but he has a great and uplifting personality and set me at ease. We also spoke about my phobia of being sick. He has prescribed some relaxation tablets to place under my tongue for the drive in.

27th May

I have been really ill since discovering I have cancer then I have felt sick every day on the lead up to my treatment. I think it is nerves.

30th May

I got my brown wig today. I love it. Uploaded pictures to fb. The woman told me to eat ice chips during chemo as it helps the taste.

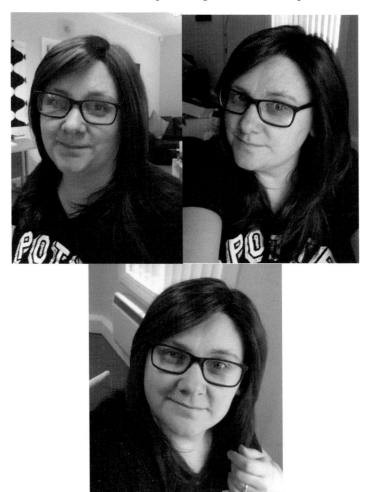

I am really scared about tomorrow.

One of the chemo nurses called me today. She informed me that this will be routine and that someone will call me the day before every chemo session to check my health. I asked her about the ice chips but she's never heard of them ever having them. She also asked if I want a cooling cap but I told her that my chemo consultant has advised against it because of the chemo in my skull. People apparently have them to stop their hair falling out. Doesn't always work but it also puts up a prevented field of the chemo getting to my skull. Not wise with the cancer in my skull too.

31st May

Chemo started. I expected to be hooked up to a drip and left alone for the duration. Instead, because of the type of cancer, a nurse has to manually pump it into my veins. It is cold and a quarter of the way through I need my arm wrapped in an electric blanket.

Before giving it to me they went through all of the possible side effects and listed all of the things I can't do or have. This basically means no take out and no sex.

Afterwards I was given lots of anti sickness meds to take home as well as moisturiser. Apparently my skin is gonna feel shitty.

By the end of the chemo, whilst the nurse is getting my prescription, I felt pressure in my nose. It was just like when your head goes under water. It was horrible. It was quickly followed by the feeling of my face having a stroke. The nurse said this is normal. My pee changed colour too. Firstly pink then orange.

Getting home that night I only needed one emergency sickness tablet but wasn't sick. Very tired though.

1st June.

Routine of sickness meds and temperature checks started. No sickness though.

2nd June.

My husband went back to work. I was grumpy. Youngest daughter checked temp whilst eldest states in bed all morning until I told her to get up. I managed my first shower and poo since chemo.

Grumpiness continued. Feeling of nausea began. Emergency sick pill taken. Went for a nap. Woke up sweating and had diarrhoea. Youngest daughter took my temp. Still within norm. Husband is anxious but I tell him to stay at work as he only has an hour to go.

7th June

I had hair cut jaw length, in preparation for losing my hair. Whilst everyone loved it I hated it. I was used to my hair being long.

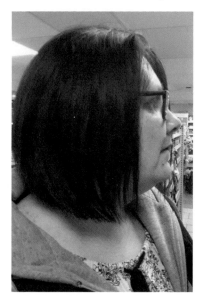

8th June

I had to go to hospital for sore throat. My white cell count had dropped to 1.65 but I was told that my throat was viral and was allowed home.

13th June

I went to Maggie's, which is a charity based on the hospital's premises to help families with cancer, for a family meeting. We made a list of questions beforehand, so we didn't forget anything. I think it made the girls feel better. Erin even got a tour of the chemo ward.

15th June

My hair started to fall out. There are no patches but my hair is thinning. I started to become self-conscious and a permanent lump formed in my throat. Still I walked around with a smile on my face.

16th June

My pubic hair started falling out and it is painful.

The pain was something I could do without but the idea of losing my pubic hair had me inwardly dancing – no ladyscaping for me, lol.

18th June

Today was my eldest's birthday and Father's day. It was a good day. In the evening I went for a shower and my hair was coming out in big clumps. My youngest came into the bathroom to brush her teeth before bed and took one look in the bath and saw all the hair and started crying. This was the final straw for me. I may not have cried in front of her, something I chose not to do because I needed to be strong for her, but inwardly it broke me.

I called my husband and told him it was time to shave my hair off.

My heart was breaking throughout it all.

19th June

My nether regions started to get sore. Not sure if it is because I had a surprise period or my hairs down there are falling out or the fact I am drying out down there. It isn't cystitis as I got checked. But it is itchy, dry and sore. Sorry for writing all of this but I was asked that when I write this could I put everything, as I have friends who care for relatives and friends with cancer and they don't really know everything that goes on as the person they are caring for refuses to talk.

On the plus side to all of this, I have an awesome Wonder Woman headscarf.

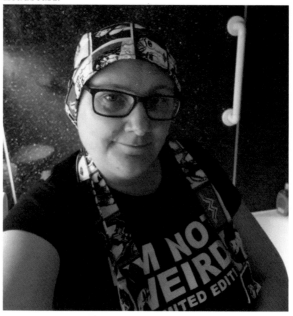

20th June

I went to something called Talking Heads at Maggie's (if I haven't mentioned before Maggie's is a charity, on the hospital grounds, that help cancer patients and their family and friends – check your hospital to see what they have.) I wasn't that keen on it but my talkative, chatty, positive side came out. There was a woman there, I would say in her twenties and she was very emotional. She has three children, the oldest being five. She was struggling with her diagnosis. I like to think that I made her smile at some point today with my randomness. I have a habit of saying weird things and the wrong times that make people laugh. I think I even mentioned being liberated by not having to shave my pubic hair.

21st June

I had my second cycle of chemo and met a lovely nurse who knows I am an author ☺ One of the first things she said was "You're the author." I blushed and nodded. Maybe it is down on my notes or something.

23rd June

My vagina is still sore.

24th June

After googling about my vagina I have come up with the fact that I have thrush. No idea why this hadn't occurred to me before. I had cystitis stuck in my head because the Dr said it was common but when I went online apparently thrush is also common in cancer patients. So this morning I popped down to the chemist to get some canesten cream. It is still itchy and throbbing but it is so much better after slathering cream on my nether regions. Let's hope it clears up fast. If come Monday and there isn't a dramatic/significant change then I will call the GP.

I woke up to a friend request from my one of my brothers. I didn't expect that. He probably only added me to be nosy and won't even speak.

First week of the chemo cycle seems to have me in tears ☹

26th June

I woke with my vision blurry.

The postman came with my order of Jamberry's from fellow author Stacey Rourke. I have been told though that I can't wear them until after chemo. They are Wonder Woman because that is how I feel.

For those who don't know, Jamberry's are foil nail stickers.

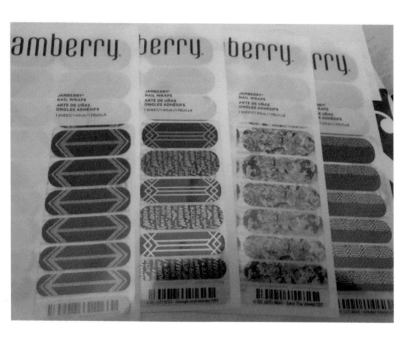

27th June

I went to the doctors in the morning to get checked to ensure that it is thrush I have. The GP believes I do and gave me medication for it and also took a swab to send away. I will only hear back if there is something else wrong.

In the afternoon I went to a group session at Maggie's called 'Feel Good, Look Good.' Or something like that. It teaches you to apply makeup. Main reason I went was to know how to do my eyebrows, which haven't fallen out yet but I want to be prepared for when they do. As a plus they give you a bag full of freebies totalling over £100. I felt like special. I got chatting to a few lovely ladies too.

28th June

I woke up to a phone call from the opticians. They had a cancellation and could fit me in before my appt on Friday. Of course I grabbed it and went along today. Before I left I had a nap and woke with a tingling sensation in my fingertips. My eyesight has drastically changed. So much so that the optician suspects that I have diabetes. Funny thing is that I have been thinking the same thing for the past two weeks with all of the drinking and peeing I have been doing. Tomorrow I am off to the GP's for 9am to have my blood taken.

Has cancer rebooted everything in my system?

I think I have piles and oral thrush. Ugh. Tried mouthwash today. Gross

29th June.

I had my bloods taken today. Apparently my bloods 3 months ago showed that my sugar levels were high. I should hear back within 5 days if I am diabetic. On another note, my daughter drew on my head. She wrote 'If you can read this I've lost my hair' then surrounded it with flowers. It was beautiful. I loved it and it was something I really wanted to do. I didn't want my whole journey to be sad and depressing, and how many times will I get to have a bald head?

30th June

I got a phone call from the Dr and they told me that the bloods I thought were taken three months ago were in fact taken three weeks ago at the hospital, the night I had to go in about my throat. Anyway my glucose was 20 then, which is really high. My fasting bloods from yesterday was 18.6. The GP said that they need to see me asap. I rushed down. First I gave a pee sample and that was fine. Then they took a finger prick test and that was 23. So I am now officially diabetic type 2. I am starting on tablets then seeing how my body responds.

1st July

I have a bloody cold sore. Ugh. Did I ever tell you that I am not a great patient. When I get a cold I act as though I have man flu. It is worse because there is not much, in the way of medication, that I can take for it.

Infection in my big toe. Hopefully I can get rid of it naturally

I watched The Secret today. I have the book but thought it would be good to retrain my mind again because obviously it has gone awry. I am a positive person and I am also thankful. I will be healthy. I am healthy ☺

2nd July

I want the confidence to sit outside, on the front step, without a head scarf on.

So I went out for two minutes and saw two people. I didn't know them but still... then I got cold and ran back in lol.

6th July

I did a take over in the Darker Side of Fiction group and I posted this picture.

Sometimes it is all about having a bit of fun. It is good to laugh.

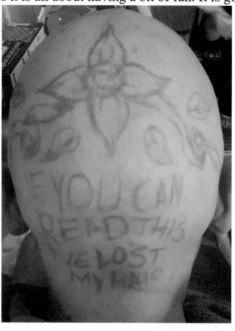

8th July

I have heard of Chicken Soup for the Soul but I didn't know they had made a Breast Cancer Survivor's one, so of course I had to order myself a copy.

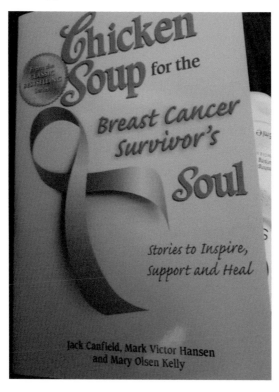

10th July

I have been tired for a few days. Today I had my bloods taken. GP called to tell me say that my white blood cell count is low.

11th July

Today I had diarrohea all day. Erin came home from my nan's.

12th July

Today I saw someone from genetics. Somehow my bloods that were taken back in May have gone missing so I need to get new blood taken for results. The hospital also phoned concerned about me having diarrohea but I assured them I was all good. Then I got off the phone and needed the toilet. Ian and I were at the beach so he had to quickly drive to Morrisons and I ended up having diarrohea. We went to the hospital and called one of the nurses outside. We spoke and decided not to have chemo today and said I can have it next week.

13th July

The hospital phoned today. I am having chemo next Tuesday 18th July at 1pm.

14th July

I got this present today from Rachel and Jo at Hourglass events. Mini eggs because… I love chocolate. Then a snitch necklace from Harry Potter. I love, love, love them.

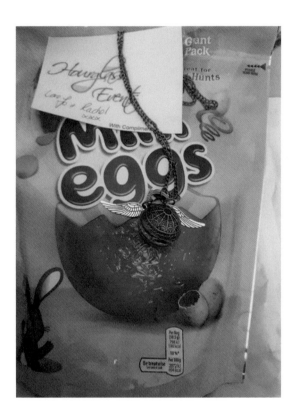

18th July

This me after today's chemo session.

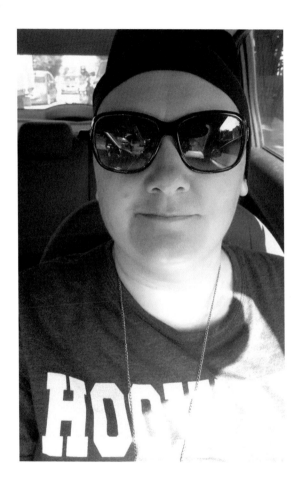

20th July

Just some of my allergies.

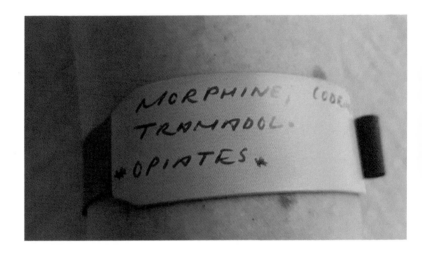

24th July

I went to have mammogram tests and the specialist told me that the cancer was almost none existent. Ian and I were so happy that we practically skipped. We decided we would keep it quiet until, only telling our daughters, until tomorrows test and not before we get it all confirmed with the dr.

25th July

I had CT scans on my chest, neck and skull today.

31st July

I saw my oncologist, Dr Hayward, today. He was running late. I wore my t-shirt that said 'I'm not weird, I'm limited edition' as well as my Harry Potter shoes. Ian and I sat in our usual place and we having fun as well as trying to decide where to go for a meal for our anniversary. Mary, the negative nurse I wasn't keen on, came over. She was lovely and asked how I am doing and offered to help get a list of all my backdated appts so I can claim back on travel expenses because it is costing us a lot. It is basically 41.5 mile round trip every time we go to the hospital and that soon mounts up.

Looking around I saw so many faces and I could instantly spot those who were going to their first appt to discover what they were going to do to treat their cancer. I saw the fear in their eyes and saw them watch me. I like to think that them seeing me wearing a wide smile helped them somewhat. Maybe this is my way of telling them to try and smile through it. There was a young girl there, maybe she was there with her parents because I did see a couple appear after an hour. But this girl was in her teens and she watched me with a smile. She even followed me to the toilets -I don't think on purpose because that would be weird lol but she was waiting outside wanting to use it.

Eventually Dr Hayward called us and said that he had some great news but we said we kind of already know. He joked it wasn't fair that someone stole his thunder, lol. He should me the letter from the mammogram specialist who said that my cancer has improved significantly in my breast, lymph nodes and chest bone. He also mentioned that there was something in the T9 section of my spine at the very beginning of my diagnosis. I didn't know this but apparently the chemo had been kicking its arse. The cancer in my skull though hadn't changed. That does not mean the chemo isn't working on it, it just means that it takes that a little longer and with the bone strengthening it will add to it.

The plan now is to have three more chemo cycles then another round of scans – not one on the skull though as they don't like doing too much radiation on the skull, which is all part of the scan. All being well that will mean that I have then put the cancer into remission and then it can be discussed how I continue my bone treatment – tablets, injections, etc. They will also give me tablets for me to take for life, a hormone blocker for sure. Because I am metastatic I will also need to have scans every 3 months for life.

One final thing Dr Hayward said was to never let my guard down. I could get an infection, it could regrow, etc. Positivity helps but you should always be prepared.

Here is me before the appointment.

My Journey: Living With Metastatic Breast Cancer.

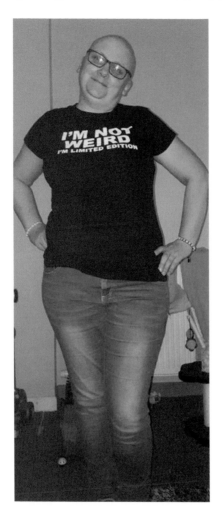

3rd August

My brother Drew and his girlfriend Jenny have come up to Scotland for a visit (yeay.) On another note, my left eyebrow has started tingling and a few hairs have fallen out. You so know that they are all going to fall out now and then grow back like a huge unibrow. I will have one giant furry caterpillar crawling above my eyes lol. Time to bring out the sharpies. I can maybe perfect my surprised look, lol.

5th August

I still keep going to run my fingers through my hair then have a 'oops' moment lol. I suppose it is like phantom limb?

8th August

The first week of chemo means small but often, when it comes to meals. It also means that I have a habit of trying things and instantly saying 'Nope, I don't want that,' before handing it off to someone else. So far this evening I have given away chocolate cake and turkey dinosaurs. I am moving on to bacon on petite pains, wish me luck.

On another note, I bought a brand new car today. Hoping to get it at the end of September. It is a Hyundai Tucson in a moon rock colour, which is supposedly a mocha colour. It just jumped out at me. #excited

Also, as it is the start of chemo again my glucose level has gone high. Thank you steroids.

10th August

In the shower and Kasey-Ray comes to see if there is anything I want.

This time I decided to answer yes. This is what I said.

"You know when I was at the hospital, the other week, getting my results? And how excited and happy I felt? Well what I want is for that to be bottled up and given to all those people who are feeling down."

She smiled and told me she loved me.

I want a charm to add to my bracelet to show the end of this battle. I want it to say 2017 not just a survivor because technically I won't fully be a survivor because my cancer is metastatic so I feel to say that I am survivor would be a lie. So this is why I want the year, this way if it does come back I can add that year as well. Each year will show the years that I kicked cancer's arse.

Went to trim up my eyebrows and realised I have lost quiet a few hairs and ones I did pluck came out pain free.

11th August

I just announced on my author page that I have cancer. You have no idea how scary that is. When I first got that page I had so much hate mail including a video showing how this person would like to kill me. FB thought that video was okay though O_o

Today I booked a gardener to come give me a quote. When Ian isn't caring for me he is working, including trying to work extra hours so we don't lose money and he is exhausted. At the beginning of my diagnosis I was told to be careful when gardening in case I got cuts etc as I can get infections easily. I have learned though that even if I wore gloves I wouldn't be able to garden for long because I get tired quickly. Not only that I find it easier to throw my back out, and that is saying something.

12th August

My husband, my rock. He doesn't normally like his picture being taken but he knows how much it means to me to make memories.

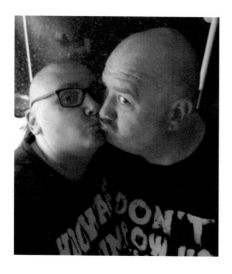

19th August

The hardest thing about the chemo treatment is definitely developing diabetes. It's no easy feat.

20th August

I hosted a charity event today, for Breast Cancer Awareness, and out of the almost forty people who said that they were definitely coming only seven people turned up. It broke my heart. I don't think people realised that. I was on an immune low week and went to all the effort to do this and hardly anyone showed. My emotions were everywhere and this just kicked me in the gut.

21st August

I was told that my monthly cycle should stop. It hasn't. It has paid a visit every single month. After chemo finishes I will be given tablets to bring on early menopause which definitely will stop my periods.

22nd August

My hands are still sore from all the needles I have had. I can still see bruises from 2 weeks and 5 weeks ago. It doesn't help that I have OCD and have to wash my hands a lot.

26th August

Lately I have days where I amuse myself by standing in front of the mirror and lifting my t-shirt. Looking in the mirror my nipples look normal. Both of them point to attention. Then I lift my arms up and giggle as my right nipple becomes inverted. It's as though it is having its own game of peek a boo.

28th August

I decided to take this picture on Snapchat and have it as my Facebook profile picture. It was a big step for me but I felt awesome.

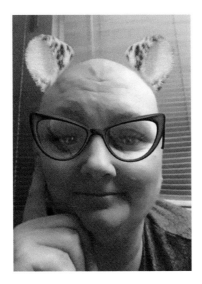

30th August

Yesterday I had my fifth session of chemo. I had left the house early as I needed to go to the Marriott hotel to see how many tables I can fit in so I know how many other authors I can invite. Anyway, whilst there my phone rang, my husband took the call, and it was ward 1 – where I have chemo – apparently there was a problem with my bloods and they and they wanted me to come in early for have another blood count. Before that I had to go and get my eyes checked as part of having diabetes. Hopefully I won't have to have it again because I am hoping that by Christmas my diabetes will have gone.

So at 1:30pm I go to ward 1 and discover that my white cell count reading, from Monday was 1.26 (or 1.2 something.) To have chemo your white cell count has to be at least 1.5. I decided to stay after the blood was taken because I was tired. Before having blood I had to go and soak my hands in hot water, to bring my veins to the surface.

As I took my bracelets off – bracelets that I only wear for chemo – one of the broke. I felt like crying. I wear only two bracelets. One says Gryffindor and the other says Courage. Both part of my Harry Potter collection. It was my Courage one that broke and in the process it hurt my heart.

As I waited to have my blood I relaxed and read. Finally, after over an hours wait, my blood results came back and I got the all clear. If they hadn't been given the clear I would have been sent home with antibiotics which would mean that my chemo would be delayed by a week. I didn't want that. But I get the all clear and had my chemo so that means, all being well, I only have one more chemo session.

According to the nurse I am a nurses dream patient ☺ I do have to say that a combination being tired and my nerves of chemo that I rambled a load of rubbish – poor nurse.

Also wanted to add that will my eyelashes thinning my eyes are constantly watering. According to the nurse it is because the eyelashes aren't there to stop it. They said that I may also be sniffly because I am losing hair in my nose too.

3rd September

The first week or two of chemo I tend to be grumpy. I lose all sense of humour and inside I want to start screaming and cursing at everyone. I don't though but as a result I also get teary because I am so angry. It isn't a nice feeling not being able to control emotions.

This morning one of my cats was sleeping across my chest – obviously the smaller one… could you imagine if my massive cat lay on my chest? Lol – and she slipped. You know what happens when a cat slips… the claws come out. One of her nails dragged right across my areola. It happened to be the cancer one and OMG did that hurt. I didn't shout at her because it was an accident but inside I was screaming.

My hair recently started growing back and it is soooo fluffy that I can't stop feeling it. I also ask my husband to feel it. There used to be a time when I used to ask him to feel my tits but now it is my head lol.

7th September

Today I received a letter from the South East of Scotland Genetic Service. On the 12th July I mentioned that I had met with someone from their team. We discussed my family's history with cancer before taking a blood sample to see if I carry the genes that are associated with breast and ovarian cancer. These are called BRCA1 and BRCA2 and they are hoping that eventually they will have a vaccine, like the cervical cancer vaccine. However, my tests results came back saying that I do not carry this gene. Now whilst I can cheer and think about that being a relief for my daughters I am looking at the bigger picture, and so are the genetics team. Yes they say that being high risk is reduced they can not rule out a genetic component due to both my personal and family history, which is that every person in my family who has died have all died from cancer. So obviously there is something that research has not detected yet. It is scary but this is what research is all about.

The human race has come a long way in the development of cancer treatment. Even treatment three years ago was so different than now and I like to think that thing will advance more in a couple of years. There is hope there. We have to believe.

On another note my daughters will now be eligible for a moderate risk breast screening from the age of thirty-five. The genetics team ask that they seek a referral to them before this time. I do remember them saying that they can be referred any time from the age of eighteen.

9th September

I have a cold. To a normal person you would just shrug your shoulders but for a cancer patient it is so much more because our immune systems are so low. I am lucky that before my cancer treatment started I was given a pneumonia vaccine and I know that soon I will be called to get the flu vaccine.

Because I am undergoing chemo I can not have anything with chemo as it brings my temperature down or something. So that means that all those cold and flu over the counter remedies are a no go for me. So I put it to Facebook and most said to have a hot toddy. I made my own version last night with warm milk, honey and port… it was disgusting. Then I had homemade bacon and vegetable soup – because I didn't have any homemade chicken, lol. Then I stuck Vicks vapour rub on the soles of my feet before putting socks on. I can't say I can tell a difference but it hasn't even been 24 hours yet.

12th September

My hands are still sore from where the chemo was injected going back 6 to 9 weeks. So last night I was in bed when I got the normal pain in my left hand from a needle near my thumb joint. This particular chemo session was painful where the needle went in. It was uncomfortable but the pain wasn't from the chemo but from where the needle was. Anyway, I ran my hand across the pain and noticed a small lump. I was able to move the lump but it would spring back to its original place. After fifteen minutes I went through to the living room to show my husband. He has suggested that it may be gristle (or something like that.) He explained that it could possibly be scar tissue that has built under the skin and I should phone the hospital today. I forgot. My intention was to call one of my nurses and ask them if this is normal. I must remember to do this tomorrow.

13th September

I spoke to one of my nurses today. She thinks that it could be scar tissue and as it isn't enflamed or the skin isn't broken etc. then I will be fine until I go to ward 1 next week to have chemo. She suggests that I mention it to them so they can see it.

Today I also fixed my Harry Potter bracelets ☺ I am still going to wear the ones I got from the lovely Louise Mckie, because that really touched my heart that she made them for me after I was so upset after my ones broke.

My youngest daughter asked me today if I found quitting smoking hard. Out of all the times I have quit smoking there have been three times that were extremely easy and they were through both pregnancies and when I discovered I had cancer. Other smokers don't bother me though. I can be around them without gagging or craving. Have there been times when I fancied a cigarette? Yes and I can honestly say that it has only ever been once but I was able to stamp on that thought within seconds. I vape though so I suppose that helps. I didn't through my pregnancies because I am not even sure if vaping was a thing. As I write this though it makes me think. Yes I found it easier to quit during the pregnancies because there was life growing inside me and I did not want my choices affecting them but this time is kind of different. I had that confliction of 'well I already have cancer, so…' Stupid thoughts I know. I do admit that I hate seeing cancer patients smoking. I see so many outside the hospital, hooked up to IV's and such, with a smoke in their mouths. It drives me crazy and I wanted to shout at them. My husband has said something like I shouldn't think that way. It is hard though.

14th September

The biggest thing I struggle with is fatigue. I've probably mentioned it previously but when you have the fatigue from your body's reaction to treatment on top of fatigue from both fibromyalgia and diabetes it can be hard. A lot of days I refuse to go for a nap during the day. Other days I really can't fight it. Today was one of these days.

It feels as though I haven't had sleep in a few days. I walk around with my head in this invisible bubble. People talk to me and I either don't hear or grasp what they saying or just nod and/or saying a word here or there. I get this tunnel vision. My head feels as though it is swimming.

Today was one of these days and I fell asleep within minutes and didn't wake until around 7pm.

15th September

The financial burden of having cancer is something that is there but not talked about. As an author I have struggled to write, because my mind has been elsewhere. I do try my best to write a little each night but sometimes that is difficult. Then there is my husband. He has been taking a lot of time off due to caring for me. It is horrible having to go through cancer then have the extra burden of worrying about money and feeling guilty that this is your fault, somehow. Even though I never asked to get cancer but you still feel responsible and I hate thinking these negative thoughts.

16th September

They warned me at the beginning of dry skin and such and they were right. The skin on my face is so dry that I have to just touch it and the skin falls away. Thankfully they gave me lots of moisturiser.

18th September

Tomorrow is a big day for me and I am nervous. I will continue being nervous until the 9th October.

It is written down that tomorrow is my last chemo day. I keep saying 'hopefully' as I don't want to let my guard down but my husband and nurses keep telling me that 'no it WILL be my last one.'

2nd October I will have a series of tests then on the 9th October I will get my results and be told if I am in remission or not.

So you can understand why I am feeling so nervous.

My eyes watering is making me really angry. I know it is down to the fact that I have less eyelashes but my eyes are constantly watering and my eyelashes aren't there to catch the liquid so I am wiping it away and it is starting to get sore.

19th September

In the hospital. Arrived early to get my bloods done before chemo. Was told that even though to get a full blood takes an hour it takes two hours for the kidney function test. So as my husband and youngest daughter are away to the seaside I am sitting waiting. I'm good though. I have my kindle and reading Amnesia by Cambria Hebert whilst listening to music on my phone, oh and writing this, lol.

I took half a lorazepam before I because I've been so nervous. Right now I am just very tired. Something about just lounging somewhere makes you sleepy.

I am also sure that on my notes it must say that I'm an author. Maybe it's there for nurses to know what to say to me. Even the newbies know I'm an author and point it out by asking if I am currently working on anything. It's nice.

My liver function was high but chemo is still going ahead. Whilst I wait I have my arm wrapped in an electric pad/blanket.

For the first time, that I can recall, there is a man opposite me having a blood transfusion. In all the times I've had chemo I don't remember seeing that happen. I thought maybe that was more for in-patients.

21st September

After chemo I'm always left with an orangey/pinky pee colour. So Tuesday, after chemo, my husband asks me a question that I have to share with you. A little gross but at the same time I reckon that there will be people who are fascinated to know.

Anyway, he asked if my poo changes colour. My reaction was to screech and squeal with a wtf before answering with a no. Of course my answer disappointed both my husband and youngest daughter, who thought it would be cool to have poo a orangey/pinky colour.

Yesterday I also made a reference to Justin Bieber. It was more in referencing one of his song titles 'Life is worth living.' It's very true. You only get one life and even though there maybe lots of bumps in the road you really have to make the most of it. Don't sweat the small stuff. Think positively. Smile, laugh and see the beauty in everything.

24th September

We have this membership where you can get into any historic place in Scotland for free. Today we decided to visit two of these places: Linlithgow Palace and Blackness Castle (apparently this one is where Outlander is filmed but having never watched it I have no idea.)

Anyway, it was a great day that left me feeling really exhausted. At one point I climbed this huge tower and actually thought I was going to pass out, when I reached the top. It was worth it though. A great sense of achievement. Plus, I got to spend quality time with my family.

On the way home I tried to nap but I am not great at napping in cars. Some people can do it but not me. Anyway, I could not get comfortable and thought that it would be great to bring the neck pillow from the house to the car. Then my husband asked if I wanted a cushion. Cue me becoming very confused until I remembered that I had kitted the new car in Harry Potter merchandise. So inside the car were three cushions in the back seat and I was able to use one.

I took this picture and it is a difficult picture for me to look at because I don't look great but this is who I am. It is what this disease has done to me and I want to share it with you.

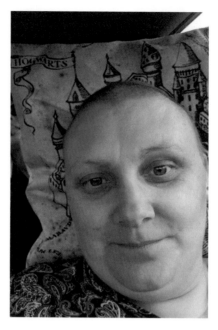

Yes I look ill but that is what I am. Funny how I still have eyebrows and eyelashes. They have thinned but I still have them ☺

25th September

I went out for a drive today. Big thing for me as I passed my driving test just before my diagnosis and haven't had the confidence or been in the right frame of mind to go out driving. I am working at it though and try and go out once a week now. It is good to have the freedom to just get out and drive but I am scared of being in control of such a lethal vehicle.

I wanted to mention weight. Before cancer I thought I would be sick all the time and lose weight. Others have suggested this too, going from experiences years ago. Before chemo started my doctor warned me to watch my weight. I was confused when he told me that I would more than likely put weight on and not lose it. He was right. Since the start I have put on two kilograms. Now here I was thinking OMG that is a lot. It is only between four and five pounds. I feel as though I have put on two stone. I can't work out because of my fibromyalgia and on top it I am more exhausted because of this stupid disease. I am hoping to try and lose weight after this battle is over.

Briefly I wanted to touch on the subject of sex. I haven't mentioned it previously in this book but it has been playing on my mind. I think it is something that needs to be mentioned. Now everyone is different but my husband and I have not made love since before my diagnosis. To me, this is probably down to me not feeling attractive. I know my husband doesn't care because he loves me for me but it is hard to feel like you want it when you are feeling less like a woman. I think losing the hair and exhaustion plays a big part in that.

27th September

I have days where anger just fills my every pore. I can feel it building days before the big explosion. It can be from people 'helping' me which makes me think that they are interfering and they think that I am incapable of doing it on my own to people not listening to my husband snoring to the arsehole neighbour who parks his company van so that it hangs over our disabled parking space. There are names for people like those neighbours and it rhymes with runt.

I can't even put this anger down to PMS because this is so much more. I was also warned about anger issues before my treatment. I just never thought I would ever feel such rage. The slightest little thing just triggers it.

2nd October

Today I went on a breakfast date with my husband. Whilst there I won a troll from one of those grabby machines. Afterwards we sat by the sea before going to the hospital for a scan of my chest and head. I'm hoping when I see my consultant next week he gives me good news. I just worry about the cancer in my skull. It hadn't shrunk on the last scan.

3rd October

Forgot to say that October is breast cancer awareness month. So go check yourself out.

6th October

Today we travelled down to Peterborough to go to my first signing since my diagnosis. I am excited. I even got to drive for over an hour on the A1(M) until my body began to protest and we had to pull into a services so my husband could take over. I am more proud with the fact that it was on the A1. It was also the longest time I had been driving at one time.

We stayed at a Premier inn and had a meal there. It was at a restaurant we had never ate in before and it was expensive and disgusting. Definitely won't be staying at that Premier inn again.

7th October

Today we got up early again. I dressed in a Wonder Woman t-shirt and head scarf as well as having Wonder Woman Jamberry nails. It was an absolutely, fantastic day. I am so glad to have been part of it. Rachel and Jo, from Hourglass Events, did a great job hosting it.

Here are just a few pictures from that day.

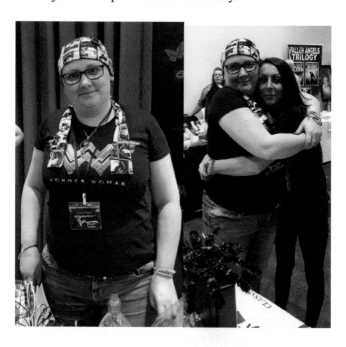

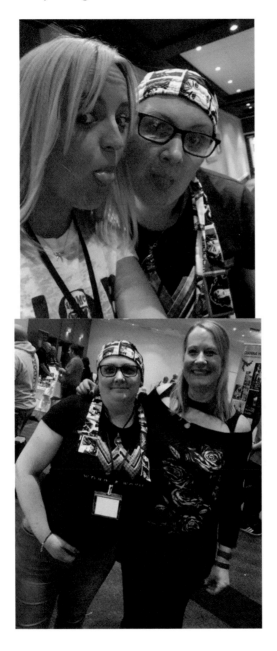

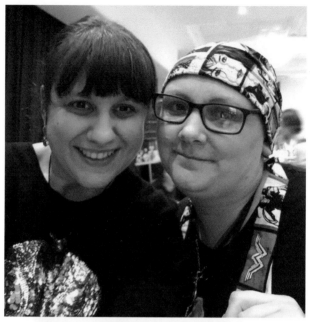

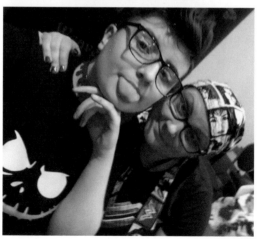

My Journey: Living With Metastatic Breast Cancer.

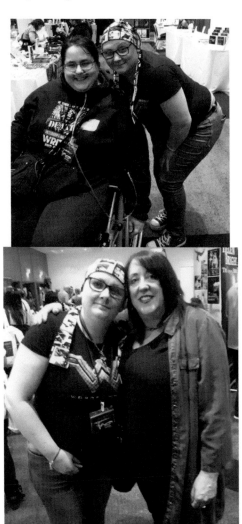

My Journey: Living With Metastatic Breast Cancer.

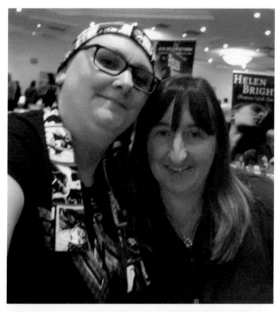

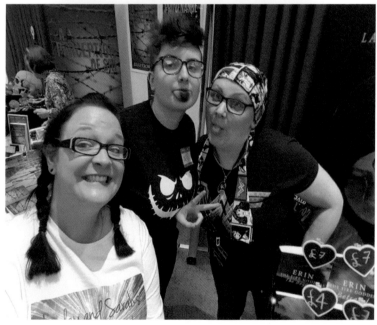

My Journey: Living With Metastatic Breast Cancer.

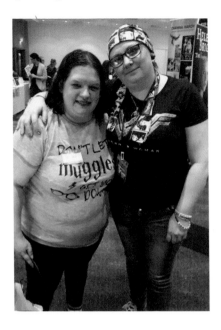

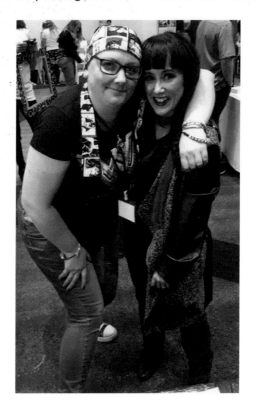

My Journey: Living With Metastatic Breast Cancer.

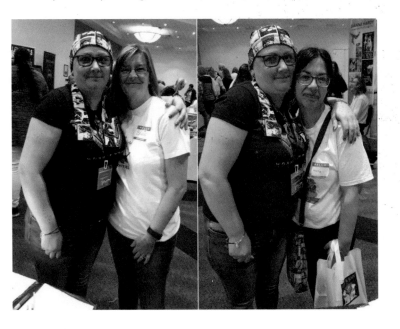

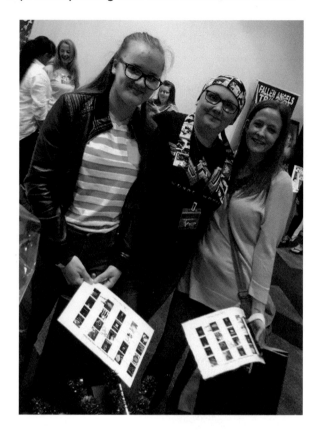

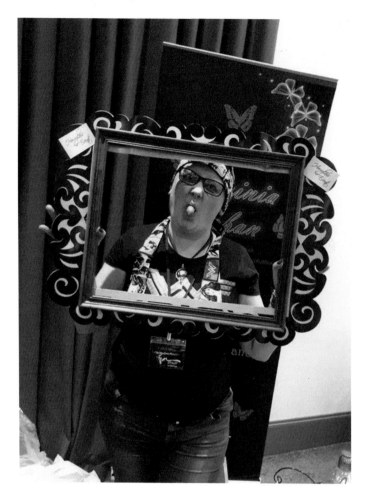

My Journey: Living With Metastatic Breast Cancer.

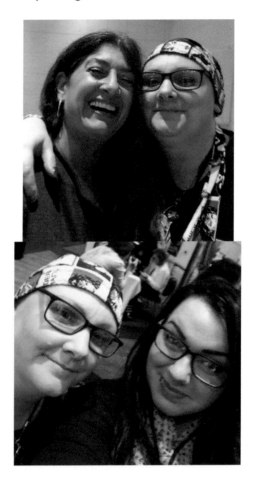

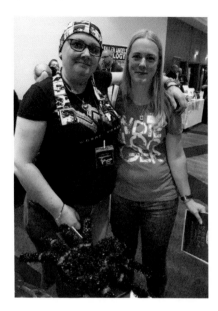

Afterwards my family and I went to get take out before going back to the Premier inn and falling asleep. It was a perfect way to end a perfect day.

8th October

Today we awoke early, yet again – I swear these early mornings are making me grumpy. I huffed and puffed – like a big bad wolf – through breakfast before we left an hour earlier than planned, mainly due to the fact that I was grumpy and wanted to leave.

We were off to my nan's home and decided to head through Melton Mowbray to see if we could buy one of their famous pies but as we approached we noticed a sign for a food festival. We had to go and investigate. All I can say is wow. The place was amazing and my husband managed to get his pies.

Finally we arrived at my nan's home. It was great to see her and soon my aunt and cousin, as well as my cousin's daughter, came to visit. They told me that I looked good and healthy. I had to tell my aunt off as she started crying which in turn made me start.

It was a great day though and I even napped in the car on the four hour journey home – I never nap in a car. Just goes to show how tired I was.

9th October

I woke up feeling both nervous and excited. I tried my best to be positive and I succeeded for the most part. The realism of the day weighed heavy on me and I was hopeful that my positivity would win out and it did but it also left me feeling confused.

So most of my cancer has shrunk immensely. The one in my skull hasn't changed so my oncologist said that this could be that the cancer is static there or it could be that it isn't cancer at all. The plan is to have scans every three months but not necessarily on my skull as the radiation can effect my head or brain… one or the two, lol.

My oncologist doesn't like to use the word remission and this is what confuses me. Do I need chemo? No but still they don't want to class it as being in remission.

Now during my whole chemo treatment I have continued getting my monthly period which means that my hormone levels are still high and this is not a good thing. So firstly I am to have something called Zoladex which is an injected to stop my periods. These will drop my hormone levels drastically and I will have this injection every 28 days for three months then after that my periods should have stopped and then they will give me other tablets to drop my hormone levels further and by then I should have started menopause – yeay… *sigh*

My bone treatment will also be changing to tablet form. I have to take one tablet every morning, at least, thirty minutes before I eat. I have to swallow it down with around two pints of water and I am not allowed to lie down as it can get stuck. (Watch as I slow blink whilst wondering wtf?)

When I left I felt overwhelmed. Do I class myself as being in remission or not? It was hard not to feel disappointed but after speaking to my husband we agreed that there is no other word for it.

I am going back to see my oncologist on the 1st December. Luckily it will be the month of Christmas so I get to wear a Christmas top ☺ By that time my periods should have finally stopped. In January is when my scans will be.

I am hopeful that things will continue to run smoothly.

Oh and I also stopped taking Gliclazide today, on my oncologists say so. He told me to call the diabetes doctor to confirm this. I did and they said it is fine and to call in a few weeks to let them know my progress.

10th October

Today I went to the GP and booked myself an appointment for tomorrow to get the injection to stop my periods – step one on the road to menopause.

Sitting here tonight and my heart feels heavy. Yesterday I may have been given, what I call, remission but I feel scared. It is metastatic. I am classed as a lifer and I am worried. I know I should just be positive and smile but it isn't that easy. I am faced with my own mortality and it scares me so much. I don't want to be negative because I feel as though it would have a negative impact on my health but it is so hard to be positive.

Maybe watching Grey's Anatomy where Maggie's mother dies from breast cancer was not the right thing to watch. I now understand why my grandparents don't like watching anything sad or with death. *Sorry for the spoiler.

11th October

I had my injection of the Zoladex implant today that will shut down my ovaries. I have this every 28 days and it swaps from side to side with each injection. Today it went in on the right side and my stomach needed to be freezed. I have numbing cream for the future ones. It is a big needle.

I also got a flu injection today.

14th October

My arm is still sore from the flu injection. I asked on Facebook how long that normally stops. Most people said a day or two then someone said that when they were on chemo it took longer.

21st October

Before my treatment my oncologist told me that I couldn't have any type of dental treatment because my treatment weekends my bones. Even though I am taking bone strengthening treatment I am sure that I will be allowed to go for a check up and scale and polish. I have so missed the dentist. I should probably double check with the oncologist to see if I can now get dental treatment, if needed.

On another note I have to say that I am happy that even though the hair on my head is growing back it isn't on my armpits and nether regions. This is great for the summer time. No idea about the legs though. I rarely ever shaved them anyway so I can't tell if it has stopped or not because I rarely ever saw hairs there.

There is also the fact that my skin is still so dry. My facial skin anyway. I am continually moisturising and putting on lip balm. It can be annoying especially if I moisturise my face at night then get up in the morning and go out only to discover that my face is dry and flaky. Most of the time I take my handbag with me and most of the time I carry moisturiser that the hospital provided. There are the odd occasions when I have nothing on me and I feel so self conscious.

At my last appointment I forgot to ask how long I am supposed to take the bone strengthening tablets and calcium tablets for.

24th October

As of today I no longer take any diabetes tablets ☺

25th October

Yesterday my mouth started feeling sore – mainly my tongue – and it has a coating on my tongue. Today I researched and it is oral thrush. I was told that I could get this during chemo typical that I get it now. Ugh

1st November

The back of my head, to the right side just below the crown, is sore. It's like a continuous throbbing sensation. Always in the same spot.

I originally started feeling this pain before I was diagnosed with cancer. Back then I put it down to a headache. Now a days I know differently. Well to a point. It has never been confirmed as cancer but there is something there in the exact place I get the pain. It worries me. I know it has neither grown nor shrunk which worries me more.

Maybe I'm worrying over nothing. But one things for sure is that I should be concentrating on writing instead of playing games.

It's like a am worrying about dying. Okay it's not like because I an always worrying about dying. Just right now I am fearful but I am stuck in this rut. A rut that I really should get out of and work my arse off writing all the books I need to write so no reader gets an unfinished series.

Maybe subconsciously I am putting it off because I think the worse won't happen for decades to come. Let's hope so because right now I worry that I will be fighting again within a year. Only this time I will probably be more tearful and angry.

8th November

I had my second injection today. I used the EMLA cream and hated it. I could feel it and have to say that I prefer just having the freeze spray.

1st December

I saw my oncologist today. He prescribed me Letrozole tablets. These are to bring my hormone levels down even further. He also said that he will be ordering scans for me. I also explained to him my fears. Throughout this whole journey I have been really positive but as soon as chemo was over I felt lost. Like I was not in control and that things could start regrowing and I would not know.

I told the oncologist that I really want them to keep checking my skull, even though they say it isn't advisable. He said he would but a couple of days after this appointment I received the appointment but there was nothing on there about the head scan. I just have to try and be hopeful.

2018

10th January

This entry is more of me checking in, so to speak. 2017 was a rough year in so many ways. My husband had to take so much time off work to help look after me that it put a dent in our finances. Yes we get free healthcare here but there are other needs such as ensuring bills are paid, housework, etc. It was a learning curve for all of us.

I am a huge overthinker so I worry about every little thing so always need distractions. Before Christmas I realised how down I was getting because our finances were stretched. I am not a depressive person but I can understand how people become depressed. At that moment I told myself off. I needed to start moping and do something about it. So I put on my positive head and start playing my positive playlist, that I played throughout chemo, and it really did change so much that a couple of days after Christmas I was fist pumping the air, after hearing some good financial news. It has made me feel really positive about the future.

Playlist

I thought I would share with you all my playlist. I picked songs with a good beat and/or a great message. For example, the Clean Bandit – Symphony made me cry when I first heard it but I love the entire thing.

- Athena Cage – All Or Nothing.
- Avicii – Wake Me Up.
- Calvin Harris feat. Florence Welch – Sweet Nothing.
- Christina Milian – When You Look At Me.

- Clean Bandit feat. Sean Paul & Anne-Marie – Rockabye.
- Clean Bandit feat. Zara Larsson – Symphony.
- David Guetta feat. Sia – Titanium.
- Ellie Goulding – Burn.
- Florence and The Machine – Shake It Out.
- Hailee Steinfeld – Love Myself.
- Jamelia – Superstar.
- Jonas Blue feat. Dakota – Fast Car.
- Jonas Blue feat. JP Cooper – Perfect Strangers.
- Justin Timberlake – Can't Stop The Feeling.
- Katy Perry – Roar.
- LL Cool J – Mama Said Knock You Out.
- Meghan Trainor – Better When I'm Dancin'.
- Meghan Trainor – Me Too.
- Meghan Trainor – NO.
- OMI – Cheerleader. (Felix Jaehn Remix.)
- Pharrell Williams – Happy.
- P!nk – Raise Your Glass.
- P!nk – So What.
- Rachel Platten – Fight Song.
- R. Kelly – World's Greatest.
- (Rocky) Survivor – Eye Of The Tiger.
- Shakira – Waka Waka (This Time For Africa)
- Sia – Alive.
- Sia – Chandelier.
- Sia feat. Sean Paul – Cheap Thrills.
- Sia – Never Give Up.
- Sia – The Greatest.
- Snakehips feat. Tinashe, Chance The Rapper – All My Friends.
- Sondr feat. Peg Parnevik – Live Love Learn.
- White Stripes – 'Seven Nation Army.'
- Wiley feat. Chipmunk – Reload.
- Yolanda Adams – I Believe.

Hair

I have struggled with my hair and feeling feminine. To some it is just hair but there are people, like me, who struggle. I love when I had long hair. It made me feel like a woman, but since losing my hair I feel more like a man. I feel like a look like a man and no matter what anyone says I do not feel attractive. So… I decided I needed to do something about it.

Firstly this is my hair now:

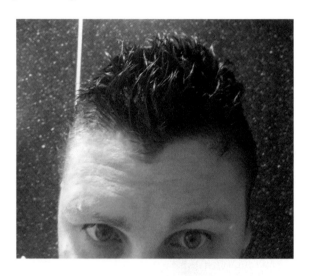

As you can see, it is getting long, but it is at that awkward stage. I do want to add that it is so thick. I mean really thick. Growing up my hair was always thin and I started using thickening shampoo that helped somewhat. When I finally did think my hair was thick I was told by numerous hairdressers that my hair was thin but there was lots of it, which is apparently different that thick hair… I don't get that, do you? Lol. I kind of get it now though because it feels so much thicker than I have ever had it.

Anyway, I want it to get long enough to be able to put it up all pretty or wear it down and straight. Right now this is not happening so I decided to get my husband to take me shopping. Bare in mine here that I am not a fan of shopping. I prefer doing it online, but if I want to feel a bit more feminine then I had to bite the bullet and go buy some hair accessories.

I want to backtrack here and mention that one of the biggest reasons for me wanting to go shopping for hair accessories is because my hair is getting longer and wearing my headscarves and going through menopause is making me boil.

So... I went shopping. Bare in mind here that I like to be different. My husband joked saying that I had said that I don't want people looking at how short my hair is but I will wear hairbands that will draw attention to it. I just shrugged.

Anyway, here are a few of the headbands I picked up.

This first one has butterflies on cat ears.

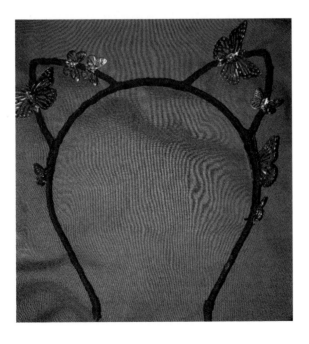

This second one is a simple headband with butterflies.

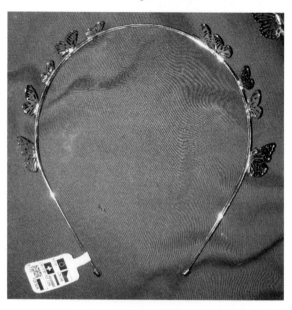

This is one of those woollen headbands, which I thought was quite apt with the snow we have been getting.

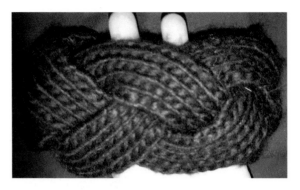

This next one I got made me so confused with how am I supposed to wear it. My automatic reaction was to put it on with the tie at the bottom, but then I was told, by my children, that I am wearing it wrong so I stand corrected, lol.

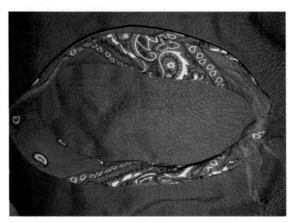

I did get more but I have put them in a 'safe' place, which basically means I have misplaced them.

MacMillan

I wanted to mention the whole MacMillan charity, because they have been amazing for me.

Now I can only talk about what goes on in the UK, anything outside then you would need to check, but if you find yourself facing the big C then I highly recommend you go see one of their financial advisors. They can help you get financial help during this tough time.

Diabetes

Christmas was tough and I had to start taking Metformin again but as things went on and having four tablets a day I felt as though I was still not getting anywhere so today I started back on Gliclazide.

I think it is time that I admitted defeat on this matter. I am a type two diabetic. The type two that can get hypos.

I have booked a telephone consultation with my GP but the earliest they have is the 24th. I told them that I will be going back on the tablets and if they have an issue then to call me.

My 2018 Outlook

After a rocky 2017 I go into 2018 with optimism.

Do I still have cancer? Yes, of course. I have metastatic breast cancer which means that it will never go away, but I am hopeful that it won't regrow for a very long time.

I plan on hitting one hundred years old and getting a letter off the King (whoever that may be then.) It is a good aim, don't you think?

Of course I want to see my children grow up and have families of their own and succeeding in whatever they choose to do.

This year though I plan on aiming to publish twelve books *gulp* Most years I aim for four but I had this crazy idea to publish twelve as a thank you to every single person out there who has been patient with me. Who has stuck by me and not asked when will my next release be. I like to think that I can do it, but if I don't well the thought was there, lol.

26th May I will also be hosting a book signing in Edinburgh. This will the first signing I have hosted and to be honest I don't think I will host another. I think it is much easier just attending events.

I will also be making two more entries in this journal – one about my scans and the other about the follow up appointment with the oncologist. Then after that it is more of a 'watch this space.' ☺

9th February

Last week I had a scan and it was hell. Not the scan itself but getting the needle put in my arm. I have never been great with needles – meaning my veins are crap.

So, the guy who called me through attempted to stick a cannula in my veins. I told him, before he had already started, that my veins are awful. I also pointed out the best vein to use – it is invisible, but it is there and a good one.

Now patients like to believe that everyone who is in charge of a bloody needle is going to be good at it. This guy was one of the worst people I have ever come across.

He could not figure out the invisible vein so decided to go for my wrist, even though I offered to stick my hands in hot water – this really helps the veins in the hand. Did he listen? Hell no. This resulted in me screaming out in pain, on more than one occasion. I was almost in tears and wanting to shout for my husband, who was waiting in the waiting room.

Finally he gave up and went to fill a surgical glove with water <insert my wtf face here>

Did he come back? No. He disappeared into the scan room and sent someone else to put the cannula in. Guess what? This person did it first time, without any issues and in the invisible vein.

Anyway, it went smoothly after that but it has mentally made me more fearful of needles.

So this brings us to today. I was nervous. So nervous. The type of nervousness that makes you want to be sick. One of the nurses told me today that this is called scanxiety… I like that term ☺

The appointment with my oncologist went well. The cancer in my skull and spine as changed. We hope this continues to remain this way.

We discussed about how my fibromyalgia is worse so I need to do some type of exercise program that will help that as well as help with the weight I have gained because of all this – steroids are hell.

Afterwards I had my blood taken by the vein whisperer – that's what my husband calls him – and that was me free to go home.

So what does the future hold for me?

I will continue to have scans every three to four months and hope that the cancer does not regrow. I know the odds are not great but I have to try and be positive even though I constantly walk around under a dark cloud of fear.

I just have to learn to live my life and put the worry at the back of my head.

All I ask is for you to send me positive vibes, but above all else I want you all to check yourselves regularly. Any slight change then please get yourselves checked out. Don't ever think that you don't want to pester the doctor or that it will be nothing. It is better to get it checked out than for it to progress and be told that there is nothing they can do.

Life is worth living. It isn't until faced with your own mortality that you realise the true extent.

About Author

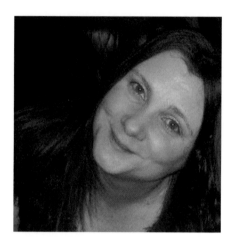

Lavinia grew up in a small town in Cheshire, England, before moving to Scotland in 2000. She now lives just outside Edinburgh with her husband Ian and their two daughters Erin and Kasey-ray. Lavinia has been writing since an early age, something that both her children have inherited. She started by writing poetry, one of which was turned into lyrics for a song. By the age of 14, Lavinia had written 7 books in an unpublished series.

After moving to Scotland she stopped writing for a while, it was only after writing a short story for her eldest daughter's school about anti-bullying and how you should stay in school and learn, that Lavinia felt the yearning to write again, this was also helped by her eldest daughter and her thirst for literature when she asked her mother to write her another story. This was how this book series came about.

Where to Stalk Lavinia

www.laviniaurban.co.uk

http://www.facebook.com/LaviniaUrbanAuthor

https://www.facebook.com/groups/LaviniasUrbanLegends

http://laviniaurban.blogspot.co.uk/

https://twitter.com/Lavinia_Missb

Lavinia is also available on Instagram, Pinterest and much more.

Printed in Poland
by Amazon Fulfillment
Poland Sp. z o.o., Wrocław